INTRODUCTION

Saxenda (liraglutide) is used for weight reduction and to assist maintain weight off as soon as weight has been misplaced, it's miles used for overweight adults or overweight adults who additionally have weight-related medical troubles. Saxenda may be utilized in kids aged 12 to 17 years who with weight problems and who have a bodyweight above 132 kilos (60 kg). Saxenda is used collectively with a wholesome diet and exercising. Saxenda is an injection given once an afternoon under the skin (subcutaneous) from a multi-dose injection pen.

Saxenda consists of the identical lively element (liraglutide) as Victoza. The difference between Saxenda and Victoza is they may be distinctive strengths and they may be FDA authorized for specific situations. Saxenda isn't always for treating kind 1 or type 2 diabetes. It is not recognized if Saxenda is secure and effective in children beneath 12 years of age. It isn't always recognized if Saxenda is secure and effective in kids aged 12 to 17 years with type 2 diabetes.

WARNINGS

The Victoza emblem of liraglutide is used collectively with food regimen and workout to deal with type 2 diabetes. Do no longer use Saxenda and Victoza together. You ought to not use Saxenda when you have more than one endocrine neoplasia type 2 (tumors on your glands), a non-public or family records of medullary thyroid cancer, insulin-dependent diabetes, diabetic ketoacidosis, or are pregnant. In animal research, liraglutide triggered thyroid tumors or thyroid cancer. It is not recognized whether those outcomes would occur in people the use of normal doses. Call your health practitioner right away when you have signs and symptoms of a thyroid tumor, inclusive of swelling or a lump for your neck, trouble swallowing, a hoarse voice, or shortness of breath.

BEFORE USING SAXENDA

You ought to not use Saxenda in case you are allergic to liraglutide, or if you have:

•   More than one endocrine neoplasia kind 2 (tumors to your glands);

•   A non-public or own family records of medullary thyroid carcinoma (a sort of thyroid most cancers); or

•   Diabetic ketoacidosis (name your health practitioner for treatment). You need to now not use Saxenda if you also use insulin or other drugs like liraglutide (albiglutide,   dulaglutide, exenatide, Byetta, Bydureon, Tanzeum, Trulicity). To make certain Saxenda is secure for you; tell your medical doctor when you have:

•	belly troubles inflicting sluggish digestion;

•	Kidney or liver sickness;

•	Excessive triglycerides (a form of fats inside the blood);

•	Heart troubles;

•	A records of issues with your pancreas or gallbladder; or

•	A records of despair or suicidal mind.

In animal studies, liraglutide induced thyroid tumors or thyroid most cancers. It isn't regarded whether or not these effects could occur in human beings using regular doses. Ask your doctor about your threat. It is not acknowledged whether or not Saxenda will damage an unborn toddler. Tell your medical doctor if you are pregnant or plan to become pregnant. It isn't recognized whether liraglutide passes into breast milk or if it is able to have an effect on the nursing baby. Tell your medical doctor in case you are breast-feeding.

Saxenda isn't FDA-accredited for use by means of everybody more youthful than 18 years antique.

WHAT HAVE TO I INFORM MY CARE TEAM EARLIER THAN I TAKE THIS MEDICATION?

They need to recognise if you have any of those conditions:

•	Endocrine tumors (MEN 2) or if a person for your family had these tumors

•	Gallbladder disorder

•	High cholesterol

•	History of alcohol abuse trouble

•	History of pancreatitis

•	Kidney sickness or in case you are on dialysis

- Liver ailment

- Previous swelling of the tongue, face, or lips with trouble respiratory, difficulty swallowing, hoarseness, or tightening of the throat

- Stomach issues

- Suicidal thoughts, plans, or try; a previous suicide try by you or a family member

- Thyroid most cancers or if a person to your family had thyroid most cancers

- An unusual or allergic reaction to liraglutide, other

medications, ingredients, dyes, or preservatives

•	Pregnant or seeking to get pregnant

•	Breast-feeding

HOW SHOULD I USE THIS MEDICINAL DRUG?

This medicinal drug is for injection underneath the pores and skin of your top leg, belly vicinity, or higher arm. You may be taught a way to put together and give this medication. Use precisely as directed. Take your medicinal drug at regular periods. Do now not take it greater often than directed. This medication comes with instructions for use. Ask your pharmacist for directions on the way to use this medicine. Read the records carefully. Talk to your pharmacist or care team if you have questions.

It is crucial which you positioned your used needles and syringes in a unique sharps container. Do no longer position them in a trash can. If you do not have a sharps box, call your pharmacist or care team to get one. A unique MedGuide may be given to you by means of the pharmacist with each prescription and top off. Be sure to read these records carefully every time. Talk for your care team approximately the usage of this medicinal drug in kids. While it can be prescribed for kids as young as 12 years of age for selected conditions, precautions do follow.

Overdosage: If you watched you have got taken too much of this medicine touch a poison control middle or emergency room without delay. NOTE: This medicinal drug is most effective for you. Do no longer percentage this medication with others.

WHAT HAVE TO I WATCH FOR WHILST USING THIS MEDICINE?

Visit your care group for normal checks on your development. Drink masses of fluids at the same time as taking this medicinal drug. Check with your care team if you get an assault of extreme diarrhea, nausea, and vomiting. The lack of too much frame fluid can make it risky with a purpose to take this remedy. This medication might also have an effect on blood sugar tiers. Ask your care group if modifications in food plan or medications are wanted if you have diabetes.

Patients and their households need to be careful for worsening melancholy or thoughts of suicide. Also be careful for unexpected adjustments in feelings along with feeling worrying, agitated, panicky, irritable, antagonistic, competitive, impulsive, critically stressed, overly excited and hyperactive, or no longer being capable of sleep. If this occurs, specifically at the start of remedy or after an alternate in dose, call your care group. Women should inform their care group if they want to grow to be pregnant or think they are probably pregnant. Losing weight even as pregnant is not cautioned and may cause damage to the unborn toddler. Talk in your care group for extra statistics.

WHAT SIDE RESULTS MAY ALSO I NOTE FROM RECEIVING THIS REMEDY?

Side consequences which you have to report to your care team as soon as feasible:

• Allergic reactions or angioedema—skin rash, itching, hives, swelling of the face, eyes, lips, tongue, fingers, or legs, problem swallowing or respiratory

• Fast or irregular heartbeat

• Gallbladder issues—excessive belly ache, nausea, vomiting, fever

- Kidney harms—decreases in the quantity of urine, swelling of the ankles, palms, or feet

- Pancreatitis—extreme belly ache that spreads to your returned or gets worse after ingesting or whilst touched, fever, nausea, vomiting

- Thoughts of suicide or self-harm, worsening temper, emotions of depression

- Thyroid most cancers—new mass or lump within the neck, ache or hassle swallowing, problem breathing, hoarseness

Side outcomes that usually do not require clinical attention (record to your care team in the event that they retain or are bothersome):

- Constipation

- Dizziness

- Fatigue

- Headache

- Loss of Appetite

- Nausea

- Upset belly

This list won't describe all feasible facet results. Call your doctor for clinical advice approximately aspect effects. You may also

document facet consequences to
FDA at 1-800-FDA-1088.

WHERE HAVE TO I KEEP MY MEDICINAL DRUG?

Keep out of the attain of youngsters and pets. Store unopened pen in a fridge among 2 and eight levels C (36 and 46 levels F). Do no longer freeze or use if the medicine has been frozen. Protect from light and excessive warmth. After you first use the pen, it is able to be stored at room temperature between 15 and 30 ranges C (59 and 86 degrees F) or in a refrigerator. Throw away your used pen after 30 days or after the expiration date, whichever comes first.

Do not store your pen with the needle connected. If the needle is left on, medicine may additionally leak from the pen. NOTE: This sheet is a summary. It won't cowl all viable information. If you have questions about this medicine, communicate on your health practitioner, pharmacist, or fitness care issuer.

HOW NEED TO I USE SAXENDA?

Saxenda is generally given as soon as in keeping with day. Follow all guidelines on your prescription label. Your physician may also from time to time alternate your dose. Do not use this medicinal drug in large or smaller amounts or for longer than advocated. Do no longer use Saxenda and Victoza together. These manufacturers incorporate the same lively component but they have to no longer be used together. Read all patient information, remedy guides, and coaching sheets furnished to you. Ask your doctor or pharmacist when you have any questions. Saxenda is injected underneath the pores and skin at any time of the day, without or with a meal. You may be shown a way to use injections at domestic. Do not self-inject this medicinal drug in case you do not apprehend the way to deliver the injection and nicely take away used needles and syringes. Saxenda comes in a prefilled injection pen. Ask your pharmacist which kind of needles is great to apply along with your pen. Your care provider will display you the excellent locations in your frame to inject Saxenda. Use a specific area each time you give an injection. Do not inject into the same place two instances in a row. Do now not use Saxenda if it has modified colours or if it has particles in it. Call your pharmacist for new medication. Also watch for signs and symptoms of excessive blood sugar (hyperglycemia) which include improved thirst or urination, blurred imaginative and prescient, headache, and tiredness. Blood sugar tiers can be stricken by stress, infection, surgical procedure, exercising, alcohol use, or skipping meals. Ask your medical doctor before converting your dose or medicine time table.

Use a disposable needle most effective as soon as. Follow any kingdom or nearby legal guidelines approximately throwing away used needles and syringes. Use a puncture-evidence "sharps" disposal container (ask your pharmacist in which to get one and a way to throw it away). Keep this field out of the reach of youngsters and pets. Saxenda is simplest part of a complete treatment software which can also include eating regimen, exercise, weight manage, ordinary blood sugar checking out, and special medical care. Follow your doctor's commands very intently.

Storing unopened injection pens: Store within the fridge. Do not freeze Saxenda, and throw away the medicine if it has grown to be frozen. Do no longer use an unopened injection pen if the expiration date on the label has exceeded. Storing after your first use: You may maintain "in-use" injection pens within the fridge or at room temperature. Protect the pens from moisture, warmness, and sunlight. Use inside 30 days. Remove the needle before storing an injection pen, and preserve the cap at the pen while not in use.

SAXENDA FACET RESULTS

Get emergency medical help when you have symptoms of an allergy to Saxenda: hives; fast heartbeats; dizziness; problem breathing or swallowing; swelling of your face, lips, tongue, or throat.

Call your doctor right now if you have:

- racing or pounding heartbeats;

- Surprising adjustments in mood or behavior, suicidal mind;

- Intense ongoing nausea, vomiting, or diarrhea;

• Symptoms of a thyroid tumor - swelling or a lump for your neck, problem swallowing, a hoarse voice, feeling short of breath;

• Gallbladder troubles - fever, top belly ache, clay-colored stools, jaundice (yellowing of your skin or eyes);

• signs and symptoms of pancreatitis - extreme pain to your higher belly spreading to your lower back, nausea without or with vomiting, rapid coronary heart fee;

• seriously low blood sugar - excessive weak spot, confusion, tremors, sweating, speedy coronary heart price, hassle talking, nausea, vomiting, fast breathing, fainting, and seizure (convulsions); or

• Kidney troubles - little or no urination; painful or tough urination; swelling in your toes or ankles; feeling worn-out or brief of breath. Common Saxenda aspect consequences can also consist of:

• Nausea (specifically while you begin using Saxenda), vomiting, belly ache;

• elevated coronary heart charge;

• Diarrhea, constipation;

- Headache, dizziness; or

- Feeling tired.

This isn't a whole list of aspect effects and others can also arise. Call your physician for scientific advice about facet effects. You may additionally document side outcomes to FDA at 1-800-FDA-1088.

WHAT OTHER PILLS WILL HAVE AN EFFECT ON SAXENDA?

Saxenda can gradual your digestion and it can take longer to your body to take in any medicines you are taking through mouth.

Tell your doctor about all of your present day medicines and any you start or forestall the use of, in particular:

• Insulin; or

• Oral diabetes medicine - Glucotrol, Metaglip, Amaryl, Avandaryl, Duetact, DiaBeta, Micronase, Glucovance, and others.

This list is not complete. Other capsules may additionally engage with liraglutide, together with prescription and over the counter drug treatments, nutrients, and herbal merchandise. Not all feasible interactions are indexed on this medicine guide.

HOW MANY SAXENDA PENS DO I NEED PER MONTH?

The quantity of Saxenda pens you'll want per month depends on your dose. Saxenda injection is available in a 3-mL pre-crammed, multi-dose injection pen which can deliver five distinct doses: zero.6 mg, 1.2 mg, 1.8 mg, 2.4 mg, and three mg. Saxenda is to be had in p.C. Sizes of 1, 3, or 5 pens. Saxenda injection pen is available in an attention of 6 mg/mL (milliliters); consequently, one 3-mL pre-crammed Saxenda pen contains 18 mg of the active drug. One percent incorporates 5

This remedy is taken by means of subcutaneous (underneath the pores and skin) injection every day, and the dose is gradually accelerated as follows:

- Zero.6 mg daily throughout week 1

- 1.2 mg every day all through week 2

- 1.8 mg day by day during week 3

- 2.4 mg each day all through week four

- three mg day by day week 5 onwards

During the dose escalation (first 4 weeks of Saxenda remedy), you'll want 2 complete Saxenda pens and 1 mL (6 mg) from the 1/3 pen. Once you're at the renovation dose of three mg Saxenda in line with day, you will inject zero.Five mL of answer daily. One Saxenda pen will last you 6 days, so that you will want five Saxenda pens according to 30 days. You ought to discard any unused medicine in a Saxenda pen after 30 days.

HOW A LOT WEIGHT CAN YOU LOSE ON SAXENDA IN ONE MONTH?

You may not word substantial weight loss on Saxenda within the first month after starting remedy. However, over the direction of 365 days, you may lose 1-2 lbs each month. If you're preliminary body weight is 230 lbs, your total weight reduction can be to the music of -9% or 20 lbs after a yr of taking Saxenda often each day. Note: Saxenda is a once-every day subcutaneous (beneath the skin) injection. Your health practitioner will start you on a low dose and slowly boom you to the upkeep dose over a period of 4 weeks.

Therefore, you can now not see a lot trade to your weight for the first few weeks. Once you're on the renovation dose of Saxenda, which is effective for weight reduction, you must begin to observe a few weight reductions. For maximum human beings, this takes place after 4-8 weeks. Clinical trials have proven that individuals who use Saxenda alongside a healthful way of life can lose, on common, five% in their body weight in 8 weeks, 7% in sixteen weeks, 8% in 24-36 weeks, and nine% in fifty six weeks.

DOES SAXENDA MOTIVE CONSIDERABLE WEIGHT REDUCTION?

Clinical trials have shown that humans can lose a clinically good sized amount of weight on Saxenda as compared to sufferers taking a placebo (inactive drug). One take a look at sponsored with the aid of Novo Nordisk, Saxenda's maker, discovered that when fifty six weeks, the average weight reduction on Saxenda was as follows:

• Sixty two.3 % of sufferers who took Saxenda lost 5% or extra in their initial weight (approximately 12 lbs).

- 33.Nine % of sufferers who took Saxenda lost 10% or greater in their initial body weight (approximately 23 lbs).

- About 6% of patients misplaced 20% or extra in their beginning frame weight (approximately 47 lbs). This is the average weight loss with Saxenda as compared to the placebo group, as stated in a medical trial. You may lose greater or much less weight with Saxenda. Your reaction to this weight loss drug will depend upon many factors, which include consuming a healthy food regimen and getting normal bodily pastime.

If you haven't lost weight (at least four% of your beginning weight) after 16 weeks of starting Saxenda, communicate on your healthcare provider about other options.

WHAT MEALS TO AVOID WHILST TAKING SAXENDA

In general, you ought to reduce down on or keep away from these foods whilst taking Saxenda:

•	Foods high in sugar, like desserts, candies or biscuits

•	fried food

•	Immoderate alcohol

•	Foods excessive in certain fats

•	Fizzy drinks, excessive sugar strength drinks or sweetened caffeinated liquids

•	Big quantities of takeout or eating place meals

You might want to recollect slowly reducing down and thinking about what steps you can take to make the technique less difficult. For example, in case you need to cut out fizzy beverages, keep away from shopping for any on your weekly store. That way you'll prevent giving yourself the option of having a sugary drink at domestic, and you may shop having them for special events as a substitute. It's no longer continually about the styles of foods you eat, both. You ought to have in mind of your element sizes and try to limit your intake in every meal. You can retain to have three meals a day, but make each one slightly smaller. Some humans gain from ingesting little and frequently by way of deciding on to devour five smaller foods spread during the day. You can also use smaller bowls or plates when ingesting to trick your thoughts into questioning your plate is full. Remember that consuming healthily does not imply you need to absolutely reduce out on the stuff you experience consuming. Healthy consuming combines eating a balanced food regimen whilst taking part in the foods you love. If you find that you do not like a certain type of 'healthful' food, you do not have to pressure yourself to devour it. Part of growing a healthy dating with meals is to eat what you want while retaining a nutritious weight loss plan. Be conscious that one of the not unusual facet outcomes of Saxenda is hypoglycemia, additionally known as low blood sugar. Your health practitioner or pharmacist has to give an explanation for to you how to treat low blood sugar. When growing healthful meal plans, keep away from cutting out carbohydrates absolutely. You nonetheless want carbohydrates to hold a middle quantity of power in your body. If you are growing the amount of physical hobby you do, this may also lower your blood sugar. So you could need to consume barely more carbohydrates on days which you plan to exercise or be lively. Your medical doctor or dietitian will discuss a healthy eating plan with you whilst you start using Saxenda. Speak to them to find out more on how to devise your meals in a manner that helps your weight loss adventure.

THE END

www.ingramcontent.com/pod-product-compliance
Lightning Source LLC
Chambersburg PA
CBHW061313250726
48653CB00002B/923